How to Talk to Your Kid about Sex

Honesty and Openness for a Sensitive Subject

William P. Smith

New
Growth
Press

newgrowthpress.com

New Growth Press, Greensboro, NC 27401
newgrowthpress.com
Copyright © 2011 by William P. Smith.
All rights reserved. Published 2011

Cover Design: Tandem Creative, Tom Temple,
tandemcreative.net

Typesetting: Lisa Parnell, lparnell.com

ISBN-10: 1-936768-44-5
ISBN-13: 978-1-936768-44-8

Library of Congress Cataloging-in-Publication Data
Smith, William Paul.
   How to talk to your kid about sex : honesty and openness for a
sensitive subject / William P. Smith.
      p. cm.
   Includes bibliographical references and index.
   ISBN-13: 978-1-936768-44-8 (alk. paper)
   ISBN-10: 1-936768-44-5 (alk. paper)
   1. Sex instruction for children. 2. Parenting—Study and
teaching. 3. Child rearing—Religious aspects—Christianity.
I. Title.
   HQ57.S646 2011
   613.9071—dc23
                                                              2011038158

Printed in India

30 29 28 27 26 25 24 23   11 12 13 14 15

As you step out of your car at the end of the day, your nine-year-old announces that her friend Kate, standing twelve feet away, wants to be a lesbian when she grows up. Your six-year-old son wants to know how babies are made . . . and he keeps pressing for more details. Your daughter came home from seeing the sex education film at school that urged her to "go ahead and experiment" as she gets older. Your fourth-grade son has started grabbing himself and doesn't seem aware of the effect he's having on others.

To top it all off, you just learned that the elementary kids are playing Spin the Bottle on the playground with the bemused blessing of the recess aide. This sounds like way too much way too early, but you're told that *everyone* thinks it's normal. You're struggling to know how to talk about the physical aspects of relationships without sounding like you just teleported in from the 1800s.

Talk about the Context for Intimacy

In an oversexed society, it is tempting to believe that the less said, the better for everyone. That's not true. What will happen is not that your kids will hear less, but that you will have allowed everyone *except* you to shape the content of those conversations. Your children will still overhear or take part in what's said at school, on the playground, in home-school clubs, at the park, even in church. They will still be exposed to sexual content through the media, even if it's only through billboards on the highway or the magazine rack at the food store. By keeping quiet you will turn them loose into that world unprepared to handle what they encounter.

Sadly, the extent of sex education for many good church kids appears to begin and end with "Save sex for marriage." Effectively, that's like telling someone "No, no, no, no, no, no, no, no, no!" for a couple of decades, then expecting them on their wedding night to suddenly be able to say "YES!"[1]

Only slightly better is when we tell them, "God knows the way you work best, so learn to trust him in this area and just wait." Good advice, but it doesn't go far enough. It doesn't give our kids a context for why smart and sensitive people in our society come up with a completely different approach to sexuality. Simply saying that treating sexuality any other way is the result of sin is not satisfying to a thoughtful young person, especially in the face of so much pressure to accept so-called alternative lifestyles.

Here's a picture I've used to help my own kids (as well as older folks) develop a positive view of their own sexuality and organize the messages they hear from our society. It's a simple picture that gives a framework for processing ungodly messages while valuing the precious thing that our sexuality is. (As a bonus feature, you don't feel pornographic drawing it!)

I start by drawing a large circle with a smaller inner circle and say, "Context is everything. If sex [label the smaller circle for your child as you talk] is best understood within the circle of biology [label the larger circle], then it really is no different from the color of your hair.

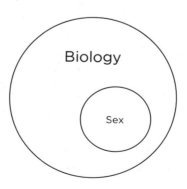

"You didn't ask for the kind of hair you have or for its color. You could just as easily have had straight instead of curly hair or red instead of brown hair and you would still be you. In fact, you can play with everything about your hair—change its color, change its style, change its length, even shave it all off—and still be you. Your personality and all the things that make up the real you will not be changed if you do different things with your hair.

"That's the same way many people think of sexuality. You got certain parts and other people got other parts. Your parts are not essential to the person you really are on the inside, so what you do with those parts doesn't change who you are either. How you use them is entirely up to you and what you do with them really doesn't make much difference.

"In a purely biological mindset, personal preference and experimentation make sense because they are simply physical aspects of a person with no necessary connection to a deeper, more essential person.

"But," I continue, drawing another set of circles identical to the first, "sex [again label the smaller circle] is much more than a piece of biology. It is better understood within the context of intimacy [label the larger circle] where it serves to connect two people at a deep level with each other.

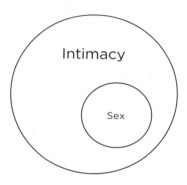

"Intimacy happens at multiple levels. There are emotional connections we build with people by the ways we share our lives with each other and the things we talk about. [Add a smaller Emotional circle within Intimacy.] In that respect, we're building intimacy between us right now. We're using words to connect our lives together.

"We also build intimacy when we do things together. [Add an Activities smaller circle.] When we go hiking or throw a ball or cook something or help shovel Mr. Gerry's driveway, we're doing something that joins our lives together.

"There are also things that people do physically that connect them; things that communicate that they like and trust each other and want to be with each other even more. People can hug each other, pat their shoulder, accidentally-on-purpose bump into each other, sit next to each other, give a back rub, hold hands, or kiss . . . or in some special cases, be involved sexually with each other. [Add labels as you talk.]

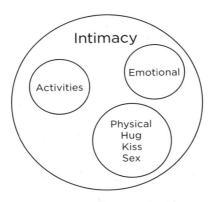

"Each of those physical expressions aims to connect two people more closely, which means you have to understand the kind of relational connection that is good for those specific people to have. A parent-child kiss is different from a husband-wife kiss because the relationship is different. Both are intimate. Both are seeking to deepen the connection they enjoy. But both are expressed differently because the goal is different. Parents and children are not trying to become one, merged life.

"God designed sex to be the most powerful physical connector, for the most special, most intimate human relationship we can have on this earth. It's the physical way you give yourself most freely and fully to someone else. It's the physical expression of two people learning to share one life (Genesis 2:23–24); it's one life lived through two bodies. It's a relationship so special and so unique that God says it is a picture of how Jesus relates to his bride, the Church (Ephesians 5:31–32). That's why God wants you only to share yourself sexually with one other person, and that should happen only when you and that person have promised to give yourselves to each other completely. That's what happens in marriage. Any other way of using sex frustrates its real purpose.[2]

"Solo flights (masturbating) don't try to connect you with anyone. Experimenting with your sexuality also misses the goal of connecting with the opposite sex at a level that reflects the sold-out-forever-only-to-each-other relationship that God shares with his bride.

"That's why we want to steer you away from sex before marriage. Since casual hookups don't try to share one life, you end up sending mixed messages. Physically you're saying, 'I am all yours and only yours' while you and the other person both know that's not true. You become a relational hypocrite. In the moment God designed for two people to be authentic and genuine with each other, you are simultaneously holding yourself back while proclaiming you're giving all you've got. You're lying.

"Everyone else recognizes you're dishonest, even if you don't, by the unflattering names they give you—playa, ho, slut, etc. The problem is worse, however, than just being insulted.

"When hooking up becomes a lifestyle, it affects the way you see people. They become things to be used and then discarded as you move on. That attitude can't be kept tightly closed in a little box. Instead, it seeps out into the way you approach friendships in general, as you teach yourself to think, 'What can I get out of this other person?' It also affects the way you see yourself, either as a user or as an object to be used by someone else. What initially looks so tempting is filled with such poison (Proverbs 9:13–18).

"Can you see how even committed couples who are sexually active but unmarried build hypocrisy into their relationship? They're willing to say something with their bodies that they're not willing or ready to say to the rest of the world: 'I promise to give you all of me now so that we literally share one life, and I will continue to do so until one of us dies.' Only when you've made that commitment and you don't care who knows it are you ready to express it physically as well. Does that make sense?"

I've found that the conversation easily moves from there as it raises other questions for your child: When should I date? How far is too far? What's wrong with homosexuality? What's wrong with Mark and Lin living together? Not easy questions, but questions that can be addressed within a relational understanding of your child's sexuality, rather than simply a biological model of personal preference, whether yours, theirs, or the broader society's.

This can't be your last conversation about sex, but it can provide a framework for a positive view of your child's developing physicality. And it pushes back against a broken world that longs to exploit it.

Practical Strategies for Change

Get Yourself Ready to Talk about Sex

In a sex-addled world, you need to prepare your child for what he will hear and see. One of the best ways to do this is to make conversations about sex and sexuality as normal and regular as anything else your family talks about. Look for those times and places where sexuality and relationships are a natural part of conversations so that you can weigh in on them. God is very concerned about sex and very explicit as he talks to you about it (see Leviticus 18, Song of Solomon, 1 Corinthians 5).

Are you ready to be as explicit as he is? You won't be able to have a good conversation if you hesitate or giggle each time you need to say "sex," "penis" or "vagina." Remember, your daughter is in elementary school; you're not. She needs to be brought into a more mature view of sex and relationships, which means you can't be more uncomfortable than she is.

This may sound silly, but if you have trouble with certain anatomical phrases, try practicing them out loud when you're alone. The more often you hear them and the more often you say them, the more natural you'll sound in a conversation. Sexuality is too important a part of any person's life for you not to learn to have regular, normal conversations about it.

Take Your Cue from Your Kids

One of the easiest ways to get started talking about sexuality and relationships is to take your kids seriously when they ask questions. Kids are naturally curious about every aspect of life. When you respond to the questions they raise, you teach them that they can trust you—that you will care about the things they care about.

I was surprised at how young each of my children were when, all on their own, they initiated a conversation about where babies came from. Inwardly I thought, *Oh wow! I didn't think we'd get to this for several more years.* But I realized that if I pulled back or looked uneasy, I would let them know that they should never feel comfortable raising that kind of subject with me again.

So I went with the flow of the conversation. I didn't volunteer extra information or suggest a next question, but I was as honest and as matter-of-fact as I could be. After a little while each one dropped the topic and we went on to something else.

I was thrilled that they asked. Part of your purpose as a parent is to help your children connect every aspect of their lives with God's way of thinking about that aspect. He urges you to bring his words intentionally into the everyday, mundane activities of life throughout the day (Deuteronomy 6:6–9). So if they're the ones asking questions, they're giving you a golden opportunity to help them understand the beauty of what God has designed. It's an opportunity you don't want to miss.

Look for Moments of Openness

Sexuality does not exist within a vacuum, but within the broader context of relationships. Therefore, your children need to have confidence in the way you handle conversations about relationships before they can trust you with something more intimate.

Many times these opportunities don't start with a direct question from your child. Instead they begin with a moment of openness when your child voluntarily shares her thoughts about relationships, inviting you to respond.

These moments come up much more frequently than you might expect, since roughly half the world is populated with people of the opposite sex from your child. He or she bumps into them all day long. These moments of openness are not always intense or of long duration, but they're another invitation from your child to weigh in on her developing sense of what relationships are supposed to be.

These moments might come as you're taking a walk with your son. He starts talking about the girl he's walking around with on the playground, or who keeps bumping his lunch tray while he's trying to eat, or who has a really exotic name, or who just moved in down the street. They might come when your daughter shares the latest sexual innuendo that a guy hopped on hormones threw in her direction. They might come while you're running football routes with your son in the back-yard. Almost in passing he pauses and tells you about someone he thinks is pretty.

Don't let such moments recede into the back-ground noise of life. Try to prolong the conversa-tion just a little by asking one question or adding one comment. Doing so tells your child that his experiences matter to you and invites him to keep sharing them.

Create Safe Spaces

Sometimes following up a moment of openness can feel risky to your child because you're asking to know him more deeply. You need to be careful at that moment to create a safe environment in which he knows you can be trusted with what he's just told you; and that you won't hurt him with what you now know.

God is like this. He knows the deepest, most closely guarded secrets of your heart and he doesn't hold them against you or use them to embarrass you. Psalm 139 makes this point. You never get the sense that the psalmist is wary of the God who sees what he does in the places that would be hid-den from anyone else's eyes (vv. 7–12). He knows that God is safe to be with. You want to help your children learn that you are safe too.

While eating dinner one night, our first grader Danny told us, "Sumita chased me at school today." Sensing a moment of openness I asked lightly, "Did you like that?" Danny gave me a quick look and hesitated just long enough for me to realize that he was making a decision about how much to trust us. He gave a little smile and said, "Yeah," then paused to see how the rest of us would respond to this new information.

I resisted the urge to tease him, said, "Cool," and kept eating. He seemed to relax, so after a little pause I asked, "So what's she like?" We proceeded to have a normal conversation about relationships.

I long for those moments—moments when my family learns to handle each other's vulnerabilities well. That context will be especially important when you talk about sexuality.

Initiate Intentional Conversations

Some kids are open and trusting while others are much more guarded. They may have reasons not to trust you or they may be more naturally closed about their thoughts and feelings. In either case, you will need to do the more difficult work of helping them get started talking.

Every Friday morning I take one of my children to breakfast before school. One of the regular questions I ask is "So, who are you hanging out with at school?" I'm happy to hear about friends of the same gender, but I want to hear about the opposite sex too. If I don't, I'll ask. I'm always careful to follow up with "And what do you like about him/her?"

Why do I start those conversations? I want to teach him that we can talk about all kinds of relationships. There are so many other people willing to have that conversation with him—his friends, songwriters and singers, movie actors and actresses, clothing advertisers, sports figures, politicians, book writers—and not one of them is shy in clamoring for his attention. I can't be either.

There's Still Hope

Are you talking about sex and relationships with your child now? If so, good, because so is the rest of society. You can judge for yourself the impact of those broader conversations on the overall health of our country's relationships.

If you haven't been, it's never too late to start. Getting started will likely be more awkward if these kinds of conversations haven't been a normal part of your friendship with your children. But the alternative to struggling through a number of clumsy, uncomfortable conversations is to surrender your little ones to the steady bombardment of the voices all around them.

Here's hope if you have to make up for lost time: if you've made it this far in this booklet, you can rest assured that you already love your children too much to surrender them to those other voices. The God who's put that kind of love in you will also give you the courage you need to make your voice heard more loudly and clearly.

Endnotes

1. My thanks to my colleague Dr. Penny Freeman for this example.

2. Timothy S. Lane's minibook, *Premarital Sex: How Far Is Too Far?* (Greensboro: New Growth Press, 2009) has a great discussion that you can share with your child of why God reserves sexual intimacy for marriage. If your child is an adolescent, you could ask him or her to read it and discuss it with you.

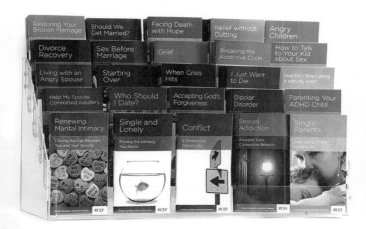